THE 5 PRINCIPLES FOR RAISING EMOTIONALLY HEALTHY KIDS

Jamie A. Garcia

Table of contents

INTRODUCTION

Do you ever think about how to raise emotionally healthy kids?

As a parent, raising kids who can control their emotions might be one of the toughest tasks, but it is necessary to remember how important this is. It is also vital to note that this will require a lot of patience, responsibility, and understanding. The purpose of parenting emotionally healthy kids is to help them build resilient, independent personalities, and equipping youngsters on how to confront the hardships of life generally from an early age helps them improve their self-confidence and self-esteem.

Who is an emotionally healthy child?
Emotionally healthy youngsters are secure in themselves and effortlessly navigate through the ups and downs of their everyday existence. They maintain healthy connections with others, manage well with stress, and keep a realistic

picture of who they are despite knowing more about the world.

PART I: GOOD PARENTING SKILL

Good Parenting

Good parenting is a wide term, spanning numerous facets of you and your child's life together. Good parenting is an accumulation of acts and interactions that you have with your kid. It is driven with purpose and ultimate objectives in mind. Good parenting tries to foster in children character characteristics including independence, self-direction, honesty, self-control, kindness, and collaboration. To that aim, successful parenting establishes a basis for a child's healthy, productive growth.

Good parenting also requires parents to live their life as role models. Kids listen to and watch what their parents do, taking everything in. As kids absorb their parents' acts and words, they begin to mimic them. Good parenting means being aware that your children are watching, learning, and copying you. Good parenting focuses on the entire health and wellness of kids. Good parenting focuses both on the here-and-now of a child's existence and on developing youngsters who are successful in their lives as they age and become adults. To that end, good parenting approaches kids with love, warmth, and acceptance. Healthy parenting entails fostering the complete kid, and attention to physical, mental, social, emotional, and intellectual needs.

A definition of excellent parenting understands that parenting is both an art and a talent. While excellent parenting doesn't imply flawless parenting (that's impossible), it does mean that parents try their best to engage constructively and react to their kids' needs every day. Every parent best differs from day to day or from hour to hour within the same day. What's vital is that a parent has a child's best interests at heart no matter what ("'Good Enough Parenting' Has Its Time and Place"). Having a child's wants and interests at heart isn't that tough when you grasp the aspects that form excellent parenting.

Good parenting entails a significant lot of regularity and routine, which provides children with a feeling of control.

Good parenting focuses on creating independence in children, therefore redundancy becomes the target for parents.
Good parenting includes a strategy that recognizes children's age and stage of development. That is, there is a fit between expectations, punishment, and resilience-building tactics with children's developmental age.

Good parenting focuses on socializing kids. Parents equip children and young people with social scripts to help them to navigate their increasing social horizons. This social scripting helps individuals navigate their online and offline lives.

Good parenting develops a growth mindset in kids rather than a mindset that says that a child's intelligence is fixed. Parenting that develops a growth mindset links kids' success to effort and strategy as opposed to purely recognizing and developing natural ability.

Good parenting focuses on encouragement over praise, consequences over punishment, and cooperation over obedience. This ensures parenting matches the times in which we live.

Good parenting urges that kids work at home without being paid so that grow to be givers, not takers.

Good parenting is nuanced to take into account children's birth order, personality, and gender differences. One parenting size doesn't fit all kids.

What Great Parents do

A Great Parent Has a Strong Marriage

"Children are affected by their parents' relationship in several ways. First, research has shown that adults who are in loving marriages are more effective parents. They're more patient and more attentive to their children's needs.

Unhappy parents, by contrast, are more inept when it comes to dealing with their children. They're inconsistent and sometimes harsh in the way they discipline. Overcome with their problems, they are unable to adequately care for someone else. But beyond that, the kind of marriage that a couple has profoundly affects the quality of the relationships that children will develop as they grow up. When kids watch their parents interact with one another respectfully, they get their first lessons on how to get along with other people. When they observe how their parents work through problems, they learn to resolve conflict. When they see their parents kiss, they feel comfortable and secure. In short, the strongest lessons children learn are from what goes on in their home, and the lessons of a good marriage will stay with them for life."

A Great Parent Finds Time for Fun

"Great parents are playful parents, ones who always remember how important it is to have fun with their kids. That doesn't mean, of course, that moms and dads need to be nonstop entertainers or amuse their kids every minute of the day. What it means is embracing the joy of a child's world and sharing it by being part of their play.

"As we sprint from one event to the next, we sometimes overlook the benefits of leisure. But simple play is immensely significant. Early games like peekaboo and hide-and-seek educate toddlers about connection. Fantasy play helps youngsters discover who they are and who they aspire to be. Playful wrestling promotes physical confidence. Tossing a ball back and forth develops athletic skills, sportsmanship, and collaboration. Play is also a method that youngsters to recuperate from life's shocks. They replicate crucial emotions with their dolls or action figures.

After getting a shot, they want to play doctor and pretend to give you a shot. This time, they're in command. "Overscheduled parents may think they don't have time for playing with dolls or building with blocks. But play can ease the stress of our busy lives. When we engage playfully with our children, we find that we suddenly have more energy and feel better about ourselves and our kids. After all, play engages us in our child's world, and what better way is there to forge a deep and lasting connection?"

A Great Parent Knows How to Say No

"Many parents find that it's tough to be firm with their children. They can't set rules. They threaten but don't follow through with consequences. 'No television for a week,' a mom may tell her child in the afternoon, only to make an exception that very night. But the fact is, if we relinquish our parental authority, we are doing a disservice to our kids.

"When children are young, they desire restrictions. They seek real rules, not rubbery ones. But by the time they reach puberty, youngsters who don't perceive their parents as authoritative figures tend to search elsewhere for a code of behavior. They frequently find it in what I call 'the second family,' the collective strength of the peer group and pop culture. Immersed in this society, nice kids act out in harmful ways. They lie without shame; they experiment with drugs and alcohol; they have sex at disturbingly early ages. They do these things because, in the world of their second family, such conduct is accepted.

"The best way to protect kids from these outside influences is for parents to assert their authority with consistency and conviction from the time their children are young. Admittedly, doing so can be confusing — for good reason. We are suspicious of being too rigid because we remember oppressive parenting ourselves or we see that it doesn't work. We are wary of showing too much understanding for fear of producing overindulged, disrespectful kids who feel entitled to say and do whatever they please.
"So what's the answer? The goal is to create a balance between giving our children comfort and empathy — and simultaneously providing structure via clear expectations of how we would want them to act. It is the continual, natural back and forth between love and restrictions that is the mark of a wonderful parent."

A Great Parent Is a Great Role Model

"Every father is eager to see his kid grow up to be responsible, empathetic, trustworthy, and kind. But teaching values isn't the same as teaching a youngster to swim, kick a soccer ball, or play the piano. Eager for straightforward directions, parents usually ask me: Will it help if I take a kid to religious services? Read tales on moral issues? Engage a youngster in community service? I tell them that such things may assist but that the true key to raising a kid with character is to be a person of character yourself. "The best way to instill values is to be a strong and present role model. A lifetime spent with a generous adult creates another generous adult.

A childhood in which material goods aren't overemphasized produces a child who understands that she can't buy everything at the mall. Parents who demonstrate genuine sensitivity to a child's feelings and needs instill in him the ability to empathize with and care for others. "Values don't emerge from a textbook or debates about abstract notions. Children learn values long before they can read about them or debate them. Rather, values are taught through the routine exchanges of daily life. If a youngster loves and respects you and your ideals, he will want to embrace them and make them his own."

A Great Parent Shows a Child, Endless Love

"Showing a kid everlasting love is at the foundation of being a wonderful parent. Fortunately, this comes easy for most parents and dads: Nature has designed us to love our children. "We show our love through affection, of course. Gushing over a baby, smothering a toddler with kisses, or offering a preteen a reassuring smile are silent ways to say 'I love you.'

We also show our love by understanding what our children need at each stage of life — and providing it for them. For an infant, that involves being a source of security; for a toddler, that means providing endless encouragement. For a school-age child, it means being an inspiring teacher of life's lessons, and for a teen, it means giving timely, judicious advice. "Above all, though, we show our love by being a steady, reliable, and attentive presence in a child's life. This requires spending quality time — and spending significant sums of time. It includes building strong family customs and appreciating idle peaceful times. No abilities in parenting substitute for a mother's and father's attentive and dedicated presence. There is nothing more commonplace — or exquisite — than being a good parent, nothing that makes us feel more vulnerable, and nothing that makes us feel more proud than knowing that, through our children, we have walked this world and made a difference."

PART II: THE 5 PRINCIPLES

Principle 1: Parenting Intentionally

Intentional parenting is a strategy for building secure, stable, and supportive parent-child interactions. Through deliberate parenting, parents and those in a parenting position create strong social and emotional abilities in their children. The intentional parenting method depends on brain research to teach you techniques to be present and active with your kid. Using the technique gives a regular framework and rules within which your youngster may discover their path. Intentional parenting employs intentional communication to approach complex challenges in a manner that enriches the parent-child bond.

Why Is Intentional Parenting Important?

Research on parenting reveals that when you as a parent or someone in a parenting position participate in particular activities, it has beneficial outcomes and encourages healthy development in your kid. Intentional parenting is oriented toward participating in various sorts of parenting practices which include:

- being attentive and involved,
- demonstrating leadership while promoting autonomy,
- having clear and predictable standards, and communicating in a manner that promotes the warmth and safety required to conduct difficult dialogues.

When certain parenting characteristics are not present or when parenting is harsh and controlling, research suggests that children experience unfavorable consequences like as; reduced emotional wellness and lack of academic accomplishment.

Studies demonstrate that when children encounter things such as harsh or abusive parenting or being in a dangerous environment, it has a detrimental influence on their brain development. This may result in mental, physical, and behavioral difficulties throughout infancy, youth, and adulthood. Intentional parenting may help you and your kid develop social and emotional skills. Put simply, social and emotional abilities comprise

- comprehending, regulating, and knowing oneself;
- relating to others; and making responsible decisions based on self and others.

Understanding oneself as a parent is one of the primary conditions for good parenting so let's start by answering these questions:

•Did you get married with the purpose of, 'I have just reached the age of marriage therefore having kids is the next step?
•Were you prepared to have a child?
•Did you ask the proper questions before you began having children?

I suppose not many of you will say yes to these questions. One of the things that I have come to learn is that many individuals were never prepared to become parents rather they all stumbled into parenthood, and simply became parents. So I can claim that parenting occurred to many of us. Understanding who you are as a parent is a major thing for good parenting. The question is, who are you? Are you able to answer this question? When I ask this question many individuals would often say that "I am a medical doctor, I am a teacher". But that's not who they are. The question of who you are is a very key and valid question that every single one of us must answer before we become parents. The major problem we have today is that we do not even understand why we became parents in the first place.

We are not aware of why we needed to be parents. We merely became parents because it was time. So as a parent, one of the things I have discovered is the position of being able to perceive, to comprehend why you are doing what you are doing. Until you understand who you are, you will keep going back and forth on your journey. One of the reasons why children are born in the world is because we are to co-create with God. I heard one of my mentors remark that "when there's an issue in the world, a kid is sent for impact. If we do not grasp that part of why we became parents is to co-create with God, then we will also miss the core of being parents and that begins from where we begin to comprehend ourselves. How much do you know about yourself?

As parents, one of the things that occurred is that we repeat what we know best. And more often than not, what we know best is through our experiences. What we know best comes from the vital part of our values, our belief system, and the things that we carry through to parenting. These are all going to come from our experiences. According to research, we all generate inferences from our subconscious and our subconscious is developed between years 0 to 7.

Everything that occurred to you when you were being parented is who you become and the lack of comprehension of who you are is what pushes us to do things against our better judgments. There is no parenting without you understanding where you come from. What are the areas that we need to look at when it comes to knowing ourselves better? What are the things that we must understand to become better parents? You cannot become a better parent without understanding a lot of the things that happened to you as a child. We can only parent better to the degree of what we know about our background, our emotional barriers, and our psychological challenges. This will determine how much we are creating a smoother or more rugged road in raising our children. "Your history, your experiences, your emotional defenses, and your psychological challenges, are deciding variables for how you will parent better now. "

What are the things that you would need to look at or you would need to discover that you need to put together in perspective when it comes to parenting your children better?

1.Self-Awareness on Parenting Ideologies:

a.Where do your thoughts on parenting originate from?

That's the first thing you want to ask yourself today. They come from how you were raised, they come from who you become, they came from your past.

Many times, I stress again and over that in parenting the reason we are to evaluate the things that the prior generation has done isn't to disparage the previous generation. It is to assist us in credit a better system for the generation to come. If we cannot examine what was done to us, then we cannot develop better as a people. So your ability to question the parenting ideologies that you already know is coming from a place of self-awareness. When you become self-aware, when you are on a path to understanding yourself, it gives you leverage over a whole bunch of other things that you believe that you know.

Other Self Awareness Questions:
b. Where do your expectations regarding children originate from?
c. What would I want to alter about my parenting today?
d. What does my kid require from me now as a parent that is different from what I needed from my parents?
e. Is it possible that I am parenting a different sort of kid from the child that I was to my parents?

2. My personality and my temperament: This is another element of you that you want to understand as a parent to be able to properly raise your kid. What are your personality and Temperament? Temperament is one of the most significant effects on your life, nevertheless, temperament is not destiny, but for you to achieve progress you need to understand that about yourself. The more you understand who you are, the more you may make adjustments that are essential in many facets of your life to become a better person. Have you been able to figure out whether you are predisposed toward being melancholy, choleric, sanguine, or phlegmatic in your behavior?

Have you ever questioned yourself, why do I behave this way because this is going to affect the sort of parent that you ultimately would become or you eventually are since now we are talking to parents and not individuals who want to become parents? Your personality is a very significant thing. Do you realize that who you have become, how you learn, and your temperament will affect how you parent children? Do you also realize that who your parents were, their temperament, and their personality influenced how they raised you? There's something that we call the parental advantage. So if your parents focused on becoming a better version of themselves, you probably had a parenting edge over the next person. Parenting advantage may put you in a better spot than your friends, merely because you had forward-thinking parents. Now the issue is, what parenting advantage would you provide your children since you were their parent?

3. Learning Style: One of the major problems I see parents have is not knowing how their children learn, but beyond that understanding how they learn. Many of us do not know how we learn. We do not know if we are kinesthetic, Auditory, or Visual learners.

So one of the major issues we have is not even that we do not understand who we are parenting, but that we do not comprehend who we are, to be able to parent who we are parenting. So you are educating your kid from your manner of learning. You do not even know what their style of learning style is, so you can truly create so much influence and advancement.

4. Emotional Awareness: You need to understand who you are emotional. A lot of people do not know how to manage emotions in any manner. How are you aware? What are you aware of when it comes to emotions? Do you know how you respond to incidences? Do you know your emotional triggers? A lot of us do not understand who we are emotionally, we are just parenting. we are simply going along and just moving. Who are you emotionally? Do you know your emotional triggers? Do you know how you react to various sorts of emotions?

5. Your growth and attachment style: There are numerous styles of attachment but the one that is at the forefront is the secure attachment style, that's the greatest. Being a parent who wants to raise a healthy kid with safe attachment, you must first be able to look within and understand your mentality, beliefs, and attachment style, as well as what caused them. Knowing yourself — making sense of your life and coming to grips with your history — is the first step in helping your children grow. Our early experiences with attachment figures are where our scripts are created. These experiences grow into basic beliefs; the mindsets, attitudes, and expectations that determine who we are, how to interact with others, and what roles we play. From before birth and well into infancy, our subconscious gets a vast quantity of data from which we create our views about ourselves, others, and the world. This is how we are trained to regard ourselves as competent or inept, decent or horrible, deserving of affection or unworthy.

Many individuals carry some degree of emotional baggage from their pasts—unhealed anguish, losses, resentments, and phobias arising from early life events. These formative experiences grow into "working models" – the underlying ideas, perspectives, and expectations about whom we are and how to interact with others. Without self-awareness, we will be dominated by these obsolete notions.

Principle 2: Parent the Child You Have, Not the One You Wish You Had

Parenting a kid who is substantially different from you might seem beyond tough. But is it a smart use of your efforts to attempt to encourage your kid to be someone different than who they are? Accepting who your kid genuinely is doesn't mean not establishing boundaries or enabling your child to be hazardous. It simply means having reasonable expectations for your unique kid and not expecting them to be someone they are not. Recommit accepting the person your kid is showing you that they are.

When you find out that you'll be raising a new kid, all kinds of notions begin to swirl about in your brain. You dream about a kid you'll have a lot in common with. As a kid, you may share the things in life that have provided you delight. You look forward to attending music recitals, and athletic activities and joyfully cheering your kid in the school play, or spending peaceful hours producing art together. Maybe you're a parent with strong political views and you can't wait to share your vision and values with the children you bring into your life.

There are simply so many plans! The clothing you'll dress your kid in, the music you'll play for them, the foods you enjoyed as a child that you can't wait to prepare for them. The tunes you will sing to them, the places you will show them. The dreams are boundless! Yep—it's all fun and games until you meet your kid in real life and you find out they have aspirations of their own!

Intellectually, you know that your kid will be their distinct personality as they grow and develop. In reality, you really can't tell ahead of time what your chemistry will be with this specific youngster. You don't know what it's going to feel like when your kid dislikes the instrument you played religiously every day after school. You don't know how much you're going to take it personally when your kid decides they want nothing to do with a topic you love and instead gravitate towards the one you struggle with. Maybe you feel shy, quiet, and studious—yet your kid is the outgoing sports-oriented class clown! So what's a parent to do? How do you learn to go with who your child is when you feel so much internal resistance when your child experiences the world in such a different way than you do?

The answer is to parent the child you have, rather than the child you might have wished to have had. Sounds easier said than done? Here are some suggestions to get you started.

Commit to being receptive to who your kid is

Whether your kid is a baby, in elementary school, or a freshman in college, you're probably not going to make it through a whole day of being with them without a few moments of emotional mismatch. You'll have difficulties calming them, understanding their wants, or loving how they behave throughout an encounter. You'll want one thing to happen and they'll desire an entirely other things!

These types of misalignments often lead to terrible fights, but they don't have to. Slow down, take a breath, and genuinely accept that, at this moment, your wants conflict with your child's needs. That in and of itself need not be an issue if you can remind yourself that you can't control who your kid is or how they think or feel. Prioritize safety requirements and attempt to let go of the rest in these situations. Focus on what is in your control: your ideas and actions. Your kid is who they are. Your kid is feeling whatever they are experiencing right now.

No amount of your irritation, disappointment, fury, and wishing it wasn't so can alter the cards you've been dealt. That useless frustration will cause you inner anguish, color your relationships with your kid, and may unwittingly convey your child the message that they aren't "good enough" for you, which causes your child inner suffering in the present and over time. Remind yourself that you can't control who your kid is or how they think or feel.

Understand, embrace, and discover things to like about your child's present stage of development

It's so hard to appreciate where your kid is in their growth without feeling compelled to push

them swiftly towards a future stage of development.
For example, as soon as a baby's legs are ready to take the least amount of weight, parents feel obliged to start having them "walk" up or down steps before they're able to accomplish this on their own. This provides newborns a false feeling of physical security that might be harmful given their real motor abilities, and parents are less present, unable to recognize the fantastic things their kid is currently accomplishing.

Don't worry too much about your future kid and some unknown development—there are so many ways that your youngster is already competent and mastered challenging abilities! Let them witness your acceptance and joy for who they already are. It's also crucial to understand your child's present stage of development so that you can have reasonable expectations about their potential. A youngster under 7 years of age is unavoidably going to have considerable trouble controlling huge emotions. Expecting a 3-year-old to manage their sadness as elegantly as a 10-year-old could is a recipe for disappointment all around!

Lean into adapting, modifying, and adjusting to your kid

If your kid had a horrible allergy to a certain food, or they were born with a particular condition or had a major accident, you would do what was required to adapt to that reality. You would avoid certain meals or seek whatever therapy your kid required or make adjustments for your damaged child while they healed. Lean into making similar accomodations for your child's emotional needs and personality.

Parents frequently attempt to make their kids be a specific way instead of making modifications around their child's temperament, personality, or even a psychiatric diagnosis. You can try to urge your child to be more outgoing, less boisterous, more academically inclined and interested in extracurricular activities, or more stereotypically masculine or feminine—but at the end of the day, your child is going to be who they are, and your relationship will be a lot smoother if you can adapt.

Reflect on how honest you were allowed to be in childhood

When you were young, were you able to show what you were feeling? Could you be honest about your animosity against your parents? Could you demonstrate sorrow, dissatisfaction, or dissent? Could you choose a sport that you enjoyed even if it was different from what your parents wanted you to take part in? Could you deny an activity if your parents wanted you to undertake it? If you were a social child whose parents were very introverted, did they support your social pursuits or shut them down? Did your parents seek to understand your interests as a teen or did they put them down or try to dissuade you from them?

Your experience as a kid will affect your comfort or unease with letting your child be who they naturally are. If your parents had a tough time embracing your actual self, such that you had to display a particular "face" to them, while being your true self in private, you could have a lot of issues accepting your authenticity as well. This could make it that much more difficult for you to let go of attempting to modify your child's natural personality. Remind yourself of what it could have been like for you to have been accepted precisely as you were, even when it wasn't easy, and even when you were having a very hard time. Remind yourself that you can offer your kid the type of acceptance that you always deserved.

Challenge yourself!

Identify the top three things about your kid that you find yourself opposing the most. Is it their interests? Their style? Their temperament or personality? A diagnosis you're having problems accepting?

Here's a challenge for the next 30 to 90 days: when you feel that old resistance to who your kid is emerging inside of you, consider radically embracing how your child is showing up at that moment. Breathe through it. Let it be. Try to swim with the stream of who your kid is rather than against it.

Accepting who your kid genuinely is doesn't mean not establishing boundaries or enabling your child to be hazardous. It simply means having reasonable expectations for your unique kid and not expecting them to be someone they are not. If your kid is high-energy and wants a lot of autonomy, you're not setting either of you up for success by placing them in circumstances where there is a lot of external control and pressure to be quiet and motionless.
Coming to grips with who your kid genuinely is may involve mourning the sort of life you hoped you'd have with your child that you—and they—will not get to experience. You may have to give up some ambitions for your child's future that they simply don't have for themselves. You may never get to share some passions or principles with your kid, and that's not easy.

Hold room for your emotional discomfort surrounding that—it's perfectly acceptable! And at the same time, day after day and moment by moment, recommit to embracing the person your kid is showing you that they are. A kid whose parent welcomes them for precisely who they are, just because they exist, is a child with a stronger ability for self-acceptance and consequently a better capacity to accept others, including the good, terrible, and ugly aspects of you, to

8 WAYS TO HONOR YOUR CHILD

Study your child

To obtain a strong comprehension of any topic, we have to study it. The same applies to every excellent connection, including our children. We need to understand what makes each of our children tick to satisfy their needs properly. What sort of personality does she have? Which learning approach appears to work best for her? If we don't take the time to discover who they are, then we will all experience irritation and misunderstanding.

Show a Genuine interest

Take a real interest in what your youngster is enthusiastic about. Spending 30 minutes playing a video game with your kid may seem like torture, but spending the time to learn about and partake in your child's hobbies can go a long way toward creating a healthy bond. Have a tea party. Play cowboys. Watch the 500th recreation of a Lego stop motion film your youngster has been producing with a grin on his face. Show your youngster that the things he enjoys are important to you.

Acknowledge their feelings

Don't belittle or disregard the way that your kid feels. Handle their sentiments carefully and with compassion. Don't make jokes or degrade them. Let your children know that how they feel is important to you. Share in their enthusiasm and excitement. Hold their hands through discouragement and despair. Be their greatest cheerleader and their biggest champion!

Find ways to say yes

If your kid has a legitimate request, find a way to say yes. Don't allow inconvenience to deprive you and your kid of chances to deepen your bond and make memories. There are lots of times we have to say no as parents, so be on the lookout for ways that you may say yes.

Keep Your word

Our children need to believe what we say to them. If you want your kid to trust you, don't create a practice of breaking your promise. I know I'm guilty of saying, "In a minute, sweetie", and it takes much longer than that to offer my attention. Being consistent is also really important.

Admit when you are wrong.

Be willing to admit when you are incorrect. Apologize, beg their forgiveness, and pray together. This will not only build your connection with your kid but also teach your youngster the appropriate approach to reconciling with others.

Give your full attention

Be engaged while you are with your children. Ask questions. Look your children in the eyes when you converse with them. Turn off your phone or at least create a phone-free time during mealtime. Our children need to know that we are listening and they have our entire attention.

Celebrate your child.

Share in your children's successes, no matter how large or little. Even if it's simply a high five and a huge grin. Let's be honest, we all like affirmation, and children need it too. Speak words of life over your children. Remember to tell your children that you are delighted they were born and that you enjoy the way God designed them.

Principle 3:Parent from wholeness instead of wound

When we are whole within, we understand and respect our existence as separate from our children's. When we are fully ourselves, we do not project on our kids—or anybody else in our relationship—any exertion of authority, any loss of power, or any uncertainty or guilt.

When we embrace and appreciate ourselves, we have clarity about life and our job as a parent. We may live out our parenting aim of unconditionally supporting and nurturing our kids. We can create and follow personal limits so we don't come in the way of our children's learning lessons and progress. We can lead and inspire while valuing and respecting our children's voices, souls, and presence. This is the only way to make room in our hearts and homes for our children to flourish.

"In the absence of reflection, history frequently repeats itself... Research has established that our children's connection to us will be impacted by what occurred to us when we were young if we do not learn to process and comprehend those experiences."

Children don't need perfection from their parents; all we need to do is avoid damaging them and provide them with the "ordinary dedication" which has always been needed of parents. But regrettably, most parents don't find this nearly so simple.

Because, first of all, there is nothing ordinary about devotion. Devotion, as parents know, is walking the floor at 2 am holding a screaming baby with an ear infection. Devotion is turning off your screens to play a board game with your kids. Devotion is forcing yourself into the kitchen to make your child dinner after a long day when all you want is to curl up on the couch and return a call to a friend. Devotion is taking off your jacket on a cold night to tuck it around a sleeping child in the back seat of the car.

This ordinary devotion is the same intense love that has caused parents throughout human history to hurl themselves between their child and danger, from flying glass to snarling wolves to enemy soldiers. But even if, most of the time, we express our devotion in our willingness to put our children first, it is still not easy to be a "good enough" parent. Because even devoted parents often inadvertently scar their children. This includes parents who adore their children, who would be completely heroic and self-sacrificing if the situation called for it. The reason is that while we would never consciously hurt our child, so much of parenting, like every relationship, happens outside of our conscious awareness.

The fact is that practically all of us were injured as children, and if we don't heal those wounds, they impede us from parenting our children optimally. If there's an area where you were scarred as a kid, you can bet on that area causing you anguish as a parent — and harming your child.

We can all think of examples: the father who unwittingly repeats his father's judgmental parenting with his sons. The mother can't set limits on her children's behavior because she can't bear their anger at her, and ends up raising anxious, self-centered kids. The parents who work long hours at their jobs, leave their babies in the care of nannies because they doubt their ability to be interested in (translate: to love) their infants.

The good news is that being parents allows us to heal ourselves. Most parents say that loving their children has transformed them: made them more patient, more compassionate, and more selfless. Loving our children helps us to heal those unloved places inside.
If we pay attention, our children have an unerring ability to show us our wounded places. Better than the best zen master or therapist, our children draw out our unreasonable fears and anger. Being parents gives us the perfect opportunity to grow and heal. Most of us run from this hard inner work, but what better motivation than our love for our children? Almost magically, as our wounds transform, we find that these hurt places inform us, motivate us, and make us better parents. And happier people.

So how can we repair our traumas, to become the parents our children deserve?

1. Parent mindfully.

If we pay attention, we discover where we're overreacting, where we need to address our own "stuff". And frankly, much of it is our crap. Not that kids don't behave like kids – they always do, and that's age appropriate. But we know that what provokes some parents would be met by others with a calm, pleasant attitude that encourages youngsters to WANT to behave – which tells us that those are our particular challenges. So every time we are "triggered," we've stumbled on something that needs mending. Seriously. Your kid understands how to press your buttons, but those buttons originate from your upbringing.

2. Break the loop by pressing your inner Pause button.

You don't have to repeat history with your kids. Even if you're already far down the wrong road, STOP. Take a deep breath, then push the pause button. Remind yourself of what is going to happen unless you select another route. Walk out of the room. Don't feel ashamed; you're demonstrating appropriate anger control. It's when you throw a tantrum that you should feel humiliated.

3. Understand how emotions function.
Anger is a biological condition. When we are in the grasp of the chemical responses that make us “angry,” we do and say things we would never choose to do otherwise. When your body and emotions are in "fight or flight" mode, your kid constantly seems like the enemy. Take a breath and wait until you calm down.

4. Reflect on your own “story.”
If you had a traumatic upbringing, you can’t alter it. But what you can alter is what you’re carrying with you from that childhood. Your “story.” You do that by meditating on it, reliving the unpleasant sensations, but also contemplating fresh viewpoints. If your father abandoned the family and you determined that you weren’t good enough, it’s time to put the record right and realize, from your mature vantage point, that you were more than enough and his departure had nothing to do with you. If your mother struck you and you inferred that you were somehow nasty within, a more true

perspective would be that your mother was afraid and would have hit even the most angelic kid in the world. You were just like any child: reaching out for affection and attention in the only ways you knew. Coming to grips with your narrative and rewriting it may be a hard process, but it's freeing. It's also the only road to becoming the parent you want to be to your kid.

5. De-Stress.

We all have a tougher time being the greatest parents we can be when we're stressed out. Develop a repertoire of habits that help you de-stress: regular exercise, yoga, hot baths, meditation. Can't find the time? Involve the entire family. Put on music and dance together, go for a stroll in the woods, put everyone to bed with books early on Friday night for a nice, pleasant evening, and catch up on your sleep.

6. Get assistance in dealing with previous difficulties.

Parenting support groups may be useful in enabling you to re-frame your parenting positively. Therapy and counseling are supposed to help you heal previous concerns and move ahead more happily in your life. There is no shame in asking for help. The humiliation comes in reneging on your obligation as a parent by injuring your kid physically or mentally. If you believe you need assistance, please don't wait. Reach out immediately.

No parent is flawless, since humans are by definition flawed. No matter how hard we work on ourselves, we will not always affect our children favorably. But if we pay attention, utilize our inner Pause buttons, reflect on our own experience, and maintain our tension at moderate levels, we may reduce the damage we inflict on our children.

Our children don't require perfection from us. Research has proven that if we address their physical, emotional, and intellectual requirements, we can typically bank on the development imperative of mother nature herself to nurture our children into fundamentally healthy individuals. And the places they're quirky? That only makes life more interesting.

Life is too brief to live in the unpleasant grips of pain, anxiety, and uncertainty. There's plenty of stuff going around. A large part of having a successful life is acquiring the fortitude to understand that being happy and loving from wholeness is not about fighting our demons, but about recognizing that there are things more essential than paying attention to them.

Principle 4: Parenting through Connection instead of correction

Meeting children's emotional needs establishes and maintains the essential link they need to flourish. The bond is a child's continuous, loving relationship with at least one other person. Studies demonstrate that many newborns and young children, in orphanages, whose physical requirements were supplied, "failed to thrive," or even died from lack of touch, attention, and connection.

Children's emotional needs are as vital as their bodily demands. Those orphans perished from non-organic failure-to-thrive because they had no constant caring relationship with at least one adult. If newborns may die from the absence of a regular loving connection, and well-attached children flourish, can that explain why children with a weak tie survive physically but do not thrive?

One of the children's most fundamental emotional demands is to be treated with respect. The basis of Connection Parenting is

treating children with respect. Children need to be treated with the same respect that we demand if we are to satisfy their desire for connection. Disrespect hurts. Hurts induce disconnection. Disconnection diminishes the strength of the parent-child bond.
For too long, children have been considered second-class citizens, as "less than"adults. The concept of treating children with the same respect we demand seems weird to parents who grew up hearing "children should be seen and not heard." many parents who grew up hearing that phrase, was questioned what it meant to them as children. . Most believe it meant that they were supposed to keep silent and how they felt or what they had to say didn't important.

Adults frequently make the mistake of assuming that, since children are smaller and have less knowledge, and less experience, they don't have the same sensations adults do. Children do have the same sentiments, and they are more fragile and vulnerable. The same words or behaviors that hurt our emotions and make us feel disrespected feel the same way to children. Dignity is not something we earn when we become adults. All of us are born with human dignity. The same words or behaviors that take away our dignity likewise take away children's dignity. One of the most prevalent criticisms I hear about youngsters "today" is that they don't treat anybody or anything with respect. How can youngsters provide respect without first receiving it? Children are not born rude; that conduct is learned. Children copy parents, family members, friends, caregivers, teachers, and television. The more children are out in the world, the more models they are exposed to. We can't keep children from ever seeing examples of the type of conduct we don't want them to mimic, but we can be more careful about which models we expose them to, particularly on television.

We cannot expect children to comprehend and implement the Golden Rule if we treat them in ways that we would not like to be treated. The proverb "what goes around, comes around;' and "what you sow, so will you reap"applies to how we treat children. It behooves any adult who seeks respect, to treat children appropriately. Whether children grow up under our roof or

not, they live in the same world we do, and their conduct affects our lives.
Most of the rude things adults say to children are so automatic, that we have already uttered them before we know it. Human beings are like tape recorders. Every word we hear is recorded forever in our minds. Adults retain "recordings" of the rude statements they heard as youngsters.

When a child's conduct pulls our buttons, our records "play" and we find ourselves repeating what we heard as youngsters. Have any parents not heard themselves repeat their parents' words to their children?
Ninety-five percent of what children learn comes from what adults model. Children are mirrors; they reflect on us everything that we say and do. Whenever adults talk, we are role models for the youngsters in our presence.

Children record every word we say to them or around them. Every time we are rude to a youngster, we are demonstrating how to be disrespectful. Children do what we do, not what we teach them to do. When we treat children with contempt, they learn to be disrespectful. We teach respect by demonstrating it and by showing them the same respect we demand. The language we grew up hearing is the language we learned to speak. Ironically, people sometimes attempt to educate youngsters to be courteous by treating them disrespectfully. When adults train children by criticizing, lecturing, humiliating, ridiculing, issuing commands, screaming, threatening, and beating, it damages children. When human beings are injured emotionally, our mind shuts down. When a child's brain is shut off, he can't learn what the adult planned to educate him to do or not to do. He can only record and replicate what is modeled.

If we are devoted to maintaining relationships with our children, we must recognize, expose, and work on eliminating treating children with disrespect. We must become the individuals we want our children to be. Treating children with respect involves a change of heart that comes only from a profound transformation in how we regard children and how we define respect.

Modeling the conduct we want children to acquire is the polite method to educate them, If we want children to have manners, to share, to apologize, to be honest, kind, respectful, and loving, we must do and be those. Learning to educate children via conscious, purposeful modeling takes time, effort, and our desire to observe and adjust our behavior. Parents are the key models in the early years. Children need caregivers who model the conduct they anticipate. When a kid doesn't act in the manner we anticipate, we ask ourselves, "Am I providing a model of the conduct I expect and will tolerate from my children?"

Remember: Our children record and mimic everything that we say and do. Learning to teach via conscious modeling is straightforward, but not easy. Stopping our old cassettes from playing is challenging. While we are educating ourselves to be as courteous to children as we are to adults, our buttons will be pressed. Our old disrespectful recordings will play and cause alienation.
We reconnect by utilizing this tool - Rewind, Repair, and Replay.

Saying, "rewind" is an indication that we caught ourselves talking rudely. We mend by apologizing. Then we repeat the event by treating the youngster respectfully. When we model repairing our conduct using rewind, repair, and replay, then we may tell youngsters to "rewind" when they speak or act in rude or inappropriate ways. They will know from our example that they, too, can reconnect by rewinding, mending, and replaying their style of speaking or behaving. When we offer children the same respect that we expect, we model respect and we sustain a connection.If we choose to tell children to be respectful by saying, "rewind" when they are rude, we must permit them to remind us to rewind when we are disrespectful.

Connecting with your kid will make your work as a parent simpler since children who feel connected listen better, feel less irritated, and adopt good actions. If your kid exhibits negative conduct, first attempt to connect with your child before addressing the problematic behavior. The conduct may be a showing of a desire for attention, feelings of abandonment or solitude, or other nasty sensations. It is also crucial to interact with your kid on a daily level, outside of the discipline. Children who feel linked to their parents have greater self-esteem, are more confident, and make better judgments. Spend at least 15-30 minutes a day connecting with your kid, with no other distractions. Let your youngster select a game or activity or perform a creative project together. Engaging in meaningful activities with your children is a fantastic opportunity to get to know them better, boost their self-esteem and character, share values, enhance emotional intelligence and make memorable memories.

Principle 5: Parent with 30 words everyday

"The way we communicate to our children creates their inner voice". This is true!
As parents, we have such a tremendous effect on the way kids view themselves. At an early age, kids believe all we say about them. And this plays a big part in growing their self-esteem and confidence! Our remarks may raise them or damage them. It's in our power to utilize our words to encourage and inspire them!

Here are some of the advantages of utilizing words of encouragement every day:

- They increase the child's self-esteem. The youngster will feel valued and respected and this will show in their level of self-esteem.
- Words of encouragement for youngsters assist them to create resilience and tenacity. A youngster who receives words of encouragement daily will be more

inclined to keep trying when things become challenging.

- These remarks will improve the child's intrinsic drive. Encouraging youngsters don't have to do with ordinary compliments and reward charts. It's about making people feel inspired and empowered to tackle problems.
- Children who routinely hear words of encouragement from their parents will also have greater confidence when it comes to facing new situations. This will help them build a growth mentality and cope easily with difficulties and failures.

I've put here a compilation of my favorite words of encouragement for youngsters. I'm sure that you already use many of them with your kids but I hope that you'll also find some nice ideas on this list.

Showing love

As parents, we presume that our kids know how much we love them. But the reality is they need to hear us say it! A simple "I love you" may improve their day!

Here are some beautiful words of encouragement for letting the tiny ones know how cherished they are!

1. I adore spending time with you!

2. Thank you for making my day so pleasant!

3. I will always adore you no matter what!

4. My life is so much better because of you!

5. You are adored.

6. I appreciate the things that we do together!

7. Thank you for making me smile every day!

8. I miss you while we are apart!

9. I am thankful to have you in my life!

Showing acceptance

One key thing that every kid has to know is that they are loved and accepted for who they are. This teaches kids that they always deserve love and respect.

10. I'm incredibly proud of you!

11. You inspire me in numerous ways every day.

12. I will always be your greatest admirer!

13. Thank you for bringing so much pleasure to our family!

14. I'm pleased to chat with you.

15. I am very delighted that you are my kid!

Building self-esteem

Showing kids affection and acceptance is crucial for helping them grow self-esteem. Here are some additional fantastic words of encouragement that boost kids' self-esteem.

16. I want to hear what you have to say about this.

17. Your opinion is always valuable to me.

18. You are a good buddy! I would have been delighted to have a buddy like you when I was your age!

19. I am extremely glad that you are such a nice and caring person!

20. You are powerful and competent!

21. You are a great person!

22. I'm intrigued to know what you think of this.

23. You're such a wonderful company!

Building confidence

Words of encouragement are also wonderful for helping youngsters establish confidence. Also, they may help them become more perseverant and robust.

24. You are such a terrific problem solver!

25. You are extremely bold when you attempt new things!

26. Mistakes are only chances to learn new things!

27. You are significant.

28. I believe in you!

29. You can make a difference!

30. Your thoughts matter.

PART III: KIDS CONFIDENCE BOOSTER

Confidence Basics

A person's confidence levels as an adult are highly affected by the degree of confidence that they had as a youngster. This is one of the key reasons why it is so crucial that you build a healthy degree of confidence in your kid. With a little bit of work and patience, your youngster will undoubtedly master this vital life skill.
There are a few things that as a parent you will need to accomplish. The following are some examples:

Always Make Time:
You must constantly make time for your kid, no matter how busy you are! Showing that your kid comes before anything else is a fantastic method of establishing a youngster's self-confidence and self-worth. It is advisable to

take the time to organize activities with your kid that might assist with the process of increasing their confidence. This may be bringing them to do something they are excellent at or maybe even getting them to try something new. This will show them that they are talented which is a terrific confidence builder. One example may be bringing a youngster to the park for a game of ball.

If your kid is not into sports, take them to an event that will enable them to exhibit their knowledge on subjects, and always be sure to convey how pleased you are.

Don't Be Too Hard:

Although it is vital not to be too soft on your kid, it is equally necessary not to be too strict on your child as well. Being overly easy on your child will likely not build good values in a kid or educate them to be responsible, on the other hand, being too difficult will likely lead to poor self-esteem since a child will feel as if they never accomplish anything right. You as a parent must find the middle ground and be equitable with your discipline. Not every kid will react to the same style of parenting so it is vital to experiment and learn what works best when it comes to growing your child's confidence.

Be a Positive Example:

It is your obligation as a parent to provide a good example for your kid and to be a role model. One of the personality qualities that your kid will certainly inherit from you is your degree of self-confidence. It is crucial that you constantly look as though you have a situation under control and that you entirely trust in yourself. Also, never speak poorly about yourself in front of your kid since this will likely induce them to start the same tendency.

Watch Out For Bullies:

Bullying is getting ever more popular. This is likely arising from the fact that youngsters may bully one another at any time and at any location, owing to social media. Bullying is arguably one of the fastest ways a child's self-confidence may be eroded. Bullies at times suffer from poor confidence in themselves, to try to make themselves feel better, they try to reduce others' confidence as well. This is why you must look out for the indicators of your kid being bullied and put an immediate halt to it! A few examples of behaviors your kid may display when being bullied are:

- Suddenly no longer wants to attend school
- Depression
- Anxiety
- Fear
- Less Social Interactions
- Not appearing Like Themselves
- Not Wanting to Talk About Their School Day

If you detect any of these indicators you need to take quick action!

Let your Child Know You Believe In Them

The second stage that we will touch base with for establishing confidence in your kid is letting your youngster know that you believe in them. This is a pretty easy procedure to complete and

involves minimal effort. However, it is still highly significant. There are numerous many methods that you may let your kid know you believe in them. With enough work and time, you will be able to identify activities that considerably boost your child's confidence while demonstrating that you believe in them.
Many individuals may be unclear about how to conduct this step efficiently and may not have a notion of where to begin. Are you one of these people? If the answer is yes do not panic, children do not come with guidebooks but you can acquire information from sites such as this book.

The process of showing your kid that you believe in them may be performed in many different ways. Oftentimes, what works for one kid will not have the same influence on another. This implies that you will likely have to test various things before you discover one that works. If you do not know where to start, a few examples are offered below:

Encourage Your Child to Try New Things:

Encouraging your kid to do new activities is a fantastic method of increasing their confidence and showing them that you completely trust in their potential to achieve anything. Pay attention to the things that your kid says to you, particularly when it comes to what they would want to accomplish but do not feel that they would be any good at it. Use this scenario as a time to demonstrate you believe in them by pushing them to attempt. Tell them that you believe in them and that they can accomplish whatever they put their mind to. It is vital to explain to children that they may not be excellent at anything when they first start but with time and with practice they will grow much better.

Push Them Out of Their Comfort Zone:

When a youngster is caught in a comfort zone their prospects of increasing their self-assurance are considerably smaller than those of a child who is continuously pushing themselves. Teaching your kid to push themselves will substantially boost their self-confidence while at the same time teaching them that you feel that they can achieve anything.

Brag about Your Child:
Bragging over your kid may be a terrific approach to increase their confidence and show them that you trust in them. This is particularly true if the boasting is done in front of them. Tell other people of their successes and the things you anticipate they will achieve in the future as this will undoubtedly improve their confidence. Do not gloat too much however since this may lead the youngster to grow big-headed.

Acknowledge Achievements and Fears

Acknowledging your kid's fears, as well as their achievements, is crucial in the function of helping your child build a healthy degree of self-confidence. This is particularly true when a youngster prevails over their fear to do something. It is crucial to remember that in trying to boost a child's confidence, every small achievement should be highlighted. No matter how minor the effort is your kid will tremendously benefit from you applauding their success.

Praise Their Achievements, Understand Their Fears

A parent's responsibility of appreciating their child's successes as well as understanding their child's concerns are two themes that we will go over in this chapter. A parent must recognize that both are equally important when it comes to the process of instilling confidence in their kid. We will go over the significance of and the methods to praise a child's accomplishments first.

Praise Their Achievements:

Praising your child's successes, no matter how minor they may appear to you, is crucial in the process of fostering confidence. This will help your kid feel good about themself and will also foster self-confidence since they will feel as though they are continually accomplishing things that amaze you. Praising your kid's successes might have more of a good consequence than continuously pointing out the bad things your child could do. This is not unexpected because continuously pointing out the incorrect thing a youngster does make them feel as though they cannot do anything right. On the other side, continually applauding your child's triumphs and not talking to them about errors that they are doing will have bad repercussions as well. This is because the youngster will feel as if they can do nothing wrong. It is crucial to establish a good balance between pointing out faults and appreciating successes.

When applauding your child's successes, you must be mindful to pamper or over-treat them. If you offer your youngster a hefty incentive every time they do a tiny job, they will naturally tend to imagine that this will happen every time they do anything. This might lead to undesirable behaviors when the incentives end since the youngster will be puzzled about why they no longer get a reward for a given activity. Prizes should be reserved for significant success. When it comes to modest successes, verbal acknowledgment or a pat on the back would satisfy just fine.

Understand Your Child's Fears:

Understanding your child's fears can play a big influence on the development of your child's self-confidence. You may be questioning, how can fear make my kid more confident in themself? The solution is the reality that conquering fear may enhance a person's self-confidence substantially. While trying to conquer phobias it is crucial that you first comprehend them. You do not want to set your kid up for failure. Some of the things they may be hesitant to undertake may truly be too tough for them. One of the worst things you can do when attempting to raise a child's confidence is to place them in a scenario where they will not win. You need to speak to your kid and find what it is that they are frightened of trying and evaluate whether it would be a good idea to push your child toward addressing those concerns. Once you understand your kid's worries and have evaluated the probable bad and good effects of addressing them, you may make the option to urge your child to face those fears. Accomplishing an activity that a youngster formerly worried they would fail is one of the finest methods to boost their self-confidence. This is because this procedure teaches kids that they can achieve things, no matter how hard they are or terrified they were if they simply set their mind to it. It is crucial to not force your youngster in to face many of their fears. Pushing your youngster too hard may result in an outcome quite different from the one you intend. It may make the youngster apprehensive which might affect the rest of their life. This might further impair their self-esteem since the fear may prohibit them from being able to perform other jobs that they could do readily at one time.

Teach Them to Learn From Errors

No one in our world is flawless therefore consequently everyone makes faults and blunders at times. The main thing is that we learn to grow ourselves and gain lessons from our failures. We must then apply these lessons to avoid ourselves from making future errors of a similar nature. It is all part of the developing process. It is the same for a youngster who needs to grow their self-confidence.

The section offers important information that will act as guidance for you when you educate your kid on the value of learning from their faults and how this connects to their self-confidence.

Help Them Learn

Your kid has been in this world far less time than you have. Therefore, it only seems fair that the task of teaching your kid how to learn from errors rests upon you. As a parent, you have had to do this many times in the past and have far more experience with it than your kid. As said previously, everyone makes errors and no one is flawless. What differentiates individuals into those who succeed and those who don't is whether a person learns from their errors or not.

Building your kid's self-confidence is attainable via achievement and success is possible through your child learning from their failures. You must educate your youngster not to be too harsh on themselves or beat themselves up when they make a mistake. You must educate them to look at the circumstance from a logical position and evaluate the things that they might have done differently to attain a better acceptable result. You will be astonished at how much this will enhance your child's self-confidence. This method will grow your child's thinking process and they will be more confident since they will know that even if they do not succeed at anything the first time, they will identify their errors, attempt again, and achieve.

Not educating your kid about learning from their errors can ultimately have detrimental repercussions on your child's self-confidence. If your kid does not learn from their errors, they will likely resume making the same mistakes. This can make a child feel as if they are stuck in a rut or like success is hopeless. They will feel like they cannot do anything and their motivation in life will slowly spiral downward. A perfect example of this would be most persons in penal facilities, whether adult or juvenile. If you ask most of the people there, they will likely say that they never had anyone teach them the value of learning from their mistakes. These people continued to make the same mistakes until they felt as if life was hopeless and completely gave up on trying to be successful. You do not want this to happen to your child. For to prevent a scenario like this, you must educate your kid on the significance of learning from their mistakes.

Learn To Accept Who Your Child Is

Accepting a kid for who they are is typically not a tough chore for a parent to undertake. On the other side, there are cases when specific traits about a kid genuinely distress their parent or parents. This may be incredibly harmful to a child's self-confidence since their parents are intended to be a source of continuing praise and love. There are some things that a kid is not able to alter about themselves and you will have to accept them if you ever want your child to be happy and have high levels of self-confidence.
This section will present you with some instances of sorts of things that parents may have to learn to tolerate. Keep in mind, some of

these things may be tough to accept or may even go against your religious background, but if you want your kid to be confident and prosper you must embrace them.

There may be some aspects about your kid that you wish could be changed. The reality is, your kid cannot alter some aspects of themself. You cannot blame your kid for who they are, they did not beg to be born into this world, and you chose to give them life. Your kid may also do some things in their life that you do not like but you must accept them as reality and seek out a method to assist your child to modify the habits. The following are some instances of sorts of things your kid cannot alter about themself.

Sexuality:

This is arguably the area where the highest number of parents have a hard time embracing their kids for who they are. This may be due to moral standpoints or it may be related to religious origins and personal views. No matter what the cause is, you must learn to accept your kid for who they are. Showing your kid that you adore them for who they are can tremendously increase their self-confidence and make them feel a lot better about themself. Apart from this, attempting to push your kid to alter anything about their self such as sexuality may bring numerous challenges for a child in life. They will most likely grow confused about who they genuinely are and this will undoubtedly harm their future and confidence.

Likes and Dislikes:
You have to learn to accept your child's likes, dislikes, and hobbies. You have to realize that just because you want your boy to grow up to be a football star or your daughter to be a beauty queen does not imply they desire the same for their lives. You need to encourage your kid to do the things they enjoy in life, even if they do not correspond to your established ambitions and objectives of your child. After all, it is their life and they are the one who has to live it, parents are merely passengers on the path used as advice.

Accept Your Child's Strengths and Weaknesses:

It is crucial for you as a parent to recognize that it may not be feasible for your kid to live up to all of your expectations. You must remember to be realistic with your expectations for your kid and to be understanding when they cannot live up to one of them. If you continuously exhibit displeasure when a youngster cannot reach one of your expectations, you will erode the child's confidence and make them feel like a lesser person or useless. Showing your kid that you would accept them as long as they do their best in all they do will raise their confidence and make them happier people with a more successful life.

These were just a few examples of the countless things you may have to accept about your child one day. As said before, you do not have to enjoy everything your kid does but you must learn how to accept it, not only for the confidence and well-being of the child but also for your own as well.

Take an Interest In Your Child's Life And Provide Opportunities For Positive Growth

While your kid is growing it is incredibly essential for you to be actively engaged in their lives and give them chances for development if you want them to be full of confidence and success. Spending time with your kid is true all that this phase demands. Do some activities with your kid that they like and utilize this opportunity to discover more about your child's life. The more you know about what is going on in your child's life the more you will be able to aid them in strengthening their confidence.

Be Involved

It is crucial that as a parent you make sure to be active in your child's life. This does not mean when it is convenient for you, it means at all times, even when tough. You may have to do things you are not interested in or attend activities that you may find uninteresting. It does not matter, you need to be involved. Being active in your child's life tells them that you care for them and at the same time improves their self-worth and self-confidence. You need to ask your youngsters questions about their lives and about how they believe things are going for them. You need to attempt to find out the areas where you can aid them to increase their confidence and create new prospects for them during these chats. A great time to do this would be during dinner, with the family eating as a whole at the dining room table and not in front of the TV on the couch.

While it is vital to go out and do activities that your kid is interested in while attempting to be more engaged with their lives, you need to make dedicated family times when the whole family spends time as a whole. This tremendously fosters the health of a family bond and makes your youngster more willing to open up to you about their lives. If your kid is honest with you they will tell you what is holding their confidence back which enables you to assist them to acquire their confidence back and be successful.

You need to take additional care to not dig into your kids' lives too closely. Trying to be overly active in your kid's life could make your youngster feel as if you are invading their lives or trying to control them. You must keep in mind that it is their life and while you may not agree with some of their actions, you have to let them develop on their own. Having a decent amount on engagement without attempting to invade your kid's life is a fantastic formula for a happy family and a confident youngster.

Why It Is Important To Provide Responsibilities

Responsibilities in life are quite crucial for a youngster, particularly when it comes to growing their confidence. You must be realistic with the duties you set for your kid since you do not want to consign them to failure. Setting obligations that are too onerous may fail which may further undermine your child's confidence. On the other side, a youngster who executes their obligations perfectly will be provided with higher self-confidence.

Set Responsibilities, Be Realistic:
While setting obligations for your kid, you must establish reasonable responsibilities. You should start with minor tasks and move up toward the bigger ones once the smaller ones can be accomplished with minimum effort.

The best fundamental duties to start with for youngsters would be chores such as cleaning their room and making their bed. After they can do this daily, you may want to begin adding extra duties such as cleaning the dishes a few times a week or vacuuming the carpet.

As a kid becomes bigger and can manage more responsibility, it is appropriate to make their obligations tougher. One suggestion that may be acceptable is getting your youngster a pet. Something smaller than a dog is suggested since most people do not know how much care a dog truly requires. It may be best to start with an animal such as a hamster or some fish. The act of having to feed this animal every day, while taking care of its other requirements, can assist your youngster to become more responsible. Properly accomplishing their obligations will also develop greater self-confidence for them because they will realize they are capable of doing tough things.
Instilling duties into your child's everyday life will be a struggle at first, but commitment and work will be beneficial in building your child's confidence.

PART IV: TIPS TO HELP YOUR KIDS THRIVE EMOTIONALLY AND MENTALLY

Have a Healthy Marriage and a Healthy You

Many people assume that mentally healthy children originate from healthy homes, while mentally sick individuals are a product of dysfunctional households, with abuse, drugs, or alcohol as a common denominator. As there are some exceptions, it makes sense that when a child's environment is healthy, they will be healthy. That being said, giving your kid what they need emotionally has a lot to do with the health of your marriage AND the well of you as a person.

Whatever you need to do to obtain it, do it. If your marriage is suffering, go to therapy. If you're battling with depression or other mental health difficulties, go to therapy and do the work required to develop individually and invest in your marriage, not just for yourself but for the well-being of your kid. You cannot model healthy for your kid if you and your marriage are not healthy.

Stay up to speed and informed of what's occurring in the world and monitor what your kids are being exposed to

Sticking your head in the sand won't do you any good when it comes to raising psychologically healthy children. What you don't know can't damage you? It can. Staying educated is among the most vital when it comes to things your kids are doing; video games, social media, current bullying concerns, societal practices, etc.

If you're not able to empathize with what they experience at school or hanging out with friends, then you won't be able to comprehend how to support them. With this information, you may remain proactive and one step ahead of things, instead of having to pick up the pieces. We can't shield kids from everything, but we can do our bit by understanding what they will confront in the world that they are growing up in.

Attend to their hearts and not their conduct

When you simply tend or handle incorrect conduct from your kid, then you presume that why they misbehaved was "just because." Sometimes, misbehavior from youngsters is, in reality, "just because." But for us to realize that we have to take the initiative and ask them questions that will help us understand why they did what they did.

If we can grasp the why, we can assist them to address their emotions, and educate them on what to deal with those that are unpleasant.

Example:

Let's assume your youngster was playing with their pal in the park, just the two of them. Then, another youngster that their buddy knew also wanted to play. Your youngster then withdraws and feels frightened by the new kid. In reaction to their fear or envy, they act out and say something harsh to their buddy. A normal reaction would be, you would confront the actions of your kid, encourage them to accept responsibility for the harm they caused their buddy, and be on your way.

But what would you be missing? Perhaps you could miss teaching them to acknowledge their sentiments of envy or intimidation. So to do this, you have to ask them—perhaps at a later time—why they did what they did, and guide them through a process of recognition and repentance, not guilt and shame.

Tell them it's perfectly normal to feel that way, and that you understand. But at the same time, direct them to the reality that acting on their sentiments caused damage, not only to their buddy but also to themselves. Help them recognize that if they act upon their sentiments of envy, it may hurt their hearts, generate bitterness, and make them sad. These are the chances we have to take to assist children to know what to do with their bad sentiments when they come. It's through these chats and times that you can fully comprehend who your kid is, and where they are coming from, which is, in essence, offering them empathy.

Deliver kids work, create rules, and give consequences "

Researchers determined that youngsters who had duties did better later in life. Chores were the greatest predictor of which youngsters were most likely to become happy, healthy, independent adults."

Make sure it's astonishingly apparent to your children that they can share their hearts with you – the good, the terrible, and the ugly.

We can't expect our children to be truthful with us when we aren't open and honest with them. Connect with your children on a personal level. Ask them questions about their day, and tell them about yours. Involve them in the tough choices you have to make at work. Tell them you got furious while driving and did something you shouldn't have and accepted responsibility for it—include them in your life so that they may learn from you.

But again, it all gets back to you. Are you healthy? Are you honest, and do you have integrity? Model for your children the attributes that represent a healthy person.

Teach them how to handle negative emotions As much as they learn to process happiness, joy, and victory, they should also learn how to handle defeat, failures, and anger in healthy ways. Never teach your kids that they should not experience unpleasant emotions and never reject they're having terrible feelings. Rather, utilize it as a method to provide a secure environment for them to recover and develop.

Admit when you're wrong and apologize Allowing your kid to experience what they need to feel, also comes the understanding of teaching them that with huge bad sentiments, come tremendous responsibilities.

We cannot manage our child's sentiments. If they are furious, they are angry—there is nothing wrong with their feeling that. But it's going a step further to teach people how to

confront their emotions, which is what we've spoken about all along.
When it comes to admitting error, the most useful method I have seen in my daughter is to acknowledge when I have mistreated her. If I am cranky and impatient with my kid, I always apologize to her after the fact—this does a few things. It tells kids that even as a parent—in their naive eyes, parents are frequently viewed as flawless—you aren't perfect, and that's good, while also demonstrating what humility is.

Humility is one of the most vital virtues you may teach your kid.
It helps individuals arrive at thankfulness, tolerate imperfection, and put others before themselves. In other words, it stops children from becoming selfish little brats. And the greatest way to teach kids humility is to exhibit it yourself.
Admission of error is one thing, but going the additional mile to say, "I'm sorry I mistreated you — you don't deserve that," is where they may, in turn, learn how to apologize to others.
In a society that is raising self-focused, narcissistic individuals, you may raise your

children to be life-givers, happy, joyous, satisfied, and thankful people. Helping kids succeed in life doesn't imply instructing them to put all of their demands and issues at the forefront of their minds—which is by common perception absurd. But by teaching children to care for others, their troubles won't seem so serious.

That doesn't imply disengaging from their difficulties and challenges, no. It is to enable people to recognize the good in the worst of a circumstance and steer them toward something positive. Directing their attention toward what they DO have, instead of what they DON'T, would help them to overcome this narcissistic world of self that we live in today.

CONCLUSION

As parents, we want the utmost best for our kids. We strive hard to produce strong people who will go on to enjoy happy lives and have excellent moral standing. Sometimes, though, we find ourselves doubting our parenting decisions, crossing our fingers, and hoping we're doing this whole parenting thing properly. Emotional awareness and the capacity to control emotions will decide how successful and happy our children are throughout life, even more than their IQ. Being an Emotion Coach to our kids has beneficial and long-lasting impacts, giving a buffer for the difficulties of life that helps them to be more confident, educated, and well-rounded persons.

Below are the dos and don'ts for growing your child's emotional intelligence.

1. Do perceive bad feelings as a chance to connect.

Use your child's unpleasant feelings as a chance to connect, heal, and develop. Children have a hard time managing their emotions. Stay empathetic, caring, and kind. Communicate empathy and compassion so that your kid may begin to grasp and put together their heightened emotional condition. Try stating, "It sounds like you're upset! I fully understand it," or, "You look so upset right now. Is it because Sandy stole your toy? I fully see why you'd be angry."

Don't reprimand, reject, or criticize your youngster for being emotional.
Negative emotions are age appropriate and will gradually fade as youngsters develop. By ignoring their sentiments as trivial or conveying the message that their feelings are terrible, you are in effect delivering the message that they are awful. This negative impression may continue with them into adulthood.

2. Do assist your youngster name their feelings.

Help your youngster give words and meaning to how they're experiencing. Once youngsters can adequately understand and describe their emotions, they're more prone to control themselves without getting overwhelmed. Try using statements like, "I can tell you're becoming upset" or, "It seems like you're truly hurt."

Don't communicate judgment or dissatisfaction.
Sometimes our kids might do or say outright inappropriate things and it's hard to grasp the feelings that seem unreasonable or nonsensical. But try putting yourself in your child's shoes. Ask questions, seek understanding, and signal to them that you're on their side, you support them, and you're there to hold their hand during those times when things seem overwhelming and stressful.

3. Do establish limitations and problem-solve.
Help them develop strategies for reacting differently in the future. Enlist their support in discovering alternate answers to their challenges. Kids crave autonomy, and this is a terrific approach to educate them that they are capable of self-regulating themselves in a world that looks unjust and especially unpleasant.

Remind them that all emotions are acceptable but all acts are not. Here's an excellent statement to establish boundaries and assist in issue solving: "I realize you're frustrated, but hitting is not appropriate. How can you express your emotions without striking next time?"

Don't underestimate your child's potential to learn and develop.
They have an inbuilt potential to evolve into high-functioning people who can problem-solve and react wisely to live's difficulties. As children, though, they need a listening ear, a hand to grasp, and a parent who can push them to reach from within and react properly.

www.ingramcontent.com/pod-product-compliance
Lightning Source LLC
LaVergne TN
LVHW052047160826
845678LV00015B/3128

* 9 7 9 8 3 5 7 4 4 0 3 5 8 *